The Formula

A health and fitness eBook guide designed to help, educate and instruct you on how to transform your mind, body and spirit.

By ELIAS NOHRA

ISBN: 9781983210440

DEDICATION

I dedicate this eBook to all my supporters who have followed me every step of the way along my journey. I hope I can use my story to propel you into creating your own.

If you wait until you're ready, you'll be waiting for the rest of your life.

CONTENTS

	Chapter	Page
1	Overcoming gym anxiety and fear of the unknown	Pg 1
2	Finding your feet	Pg 5
3	Are you an ectomorph, endomorph or mesomorph?	Pg 9
4	The Formula for fat loss	Pg 12
5	Consistency	Pg 20
6	When should I eat?	Pg 22
7	Worst substance for your body	Pg 24
8	Superfoods	Pg 26
9	Supplements	Pg 31
10	Starving yourself	Pg 36
11	Surgery	Pg 40
12	Steroids	Pg 43
13	The truth behind cardio	Pg 47
14	Mind to muscle connection	Pg 52
15	Tempo	Pg 54
16	My butt workout	Pg 56
17	My butt workout (without detail)	Pg 68

ACKNOWLEDGMENTS

Dear young Elias,

If only you weren't so hard on yourself.

PREFACE

Welcome.

You have just taken the very first step, or perhaps the next step, to being a happier, healthier, strong and more confident version of yourself. The purpose of this eBook is to present facts and statistics, offer insight and knowledge, guide you on the right path on instruct you on what you need to do in order to achieve your goals. *The Formula* will test your limits but ultimately help you obtain the physique you want. You will finally decipher what it takes to transform yourself, only if you feel it necessary. What I am about to tell you will change your life. This eBook is a guide on how to begin, continue, or find your way in a world riddled with different ways of doing things, particularly the fitness industry, or simply even, just the gym, therefore helping you to help yourself. I will guide you through your own journey by helping you create your own path.

You will also have access to my butt workout towards the end. I welcome you to skip to the very end if you are eager to find out the golden exercises, otherwise continue reading to discover *The Formula.*

1 | OVERCOMING GYM ANXIETY AND FEAR OF THE UNKNOWN

1. Find your *why* and your purpose

It is important to remind yourself the *why* as well as *what* any time you are goal setting, breaking bad habits or making a change in your life. *Why am I doing this? What do I want out of this?* Your *why* is the most important factor that will keep you going when excuses, hesitation or anxiety cloud your judgment. Think about one goal that is really important to you right now. Write down your *why* for reaching that goal and your *what* you will benefit out of it. If you can't come up with one really great answer, then create another goal.

2. Don't let what others are doing affect you

If you struggle with things like self-doubt and comparisons, write down a list of reasons why you want to better yourself. Then write down a list of reasons why the person you're comparing yourself with wants to better him or herself. You will find the reasons are usually quite similar. We are all trying to better ourselves at the end of the day. Meaning each person's journey will be similar in some way. We often get lost wondering what others are doing at the gym that it affects our training and our judgment. We are all on our own journey and path to success and greatness. You can't be great if you're in everybody else's business but your own, focusing on what they're doing and achieving, when you're not even doing what you're supposed to be doing, or achieving of what you could be achieving, which is similar to what they could be achieving. They're human too. Just like you. Find out what it is you're meant to be doing and focus on that.

3. Creating habit and routine

Putting your gym clothes on, doing your hair, spraying some deodorant or perfume, putting your earphones in, playing your favorite songs, getting into a routine with sessions; before work or after work, before class or after class, etc., are all cues to trigger a neurological 'habit loop' that helps with consistent behavior. Have your outfit planned, have your music ready, have your goals in big golden letters at the back of your mind, have what you want to achieve from your workout detailed in your thought process as you walk through the gym doors, and the routine becomes a habit. Motivation becomes intrinsic over time as the brain begins to associate increased heart rate, the burn, sweat, adrenaline and fatigue with the surge of feel-good chemicals known as endorphins, that make you feel amazing after a great workout. *Why would you let that go to waste because you're worried of someone else looking at you or what they are thinking of you?* Newsflash! They are most likely looking around at the gym and are most likely NOT concerned at all with what you are doing unless they come up to you and approach you, leading to my next point.

4. People staring at the gym

Everyone looks at everyone at the gym. It's just a fact. The sweat, adrenaline, rush, music blaring, weights slamming, hearts pounding, has everyone's mood elevated as well as their heart rate. Meaning people are going to be walking around a lot, talking (probably more than I would like them to), interacting, panting, groaning, sometimes yelling, and getting engrossed in their workout because of the feel-good feeling. They are not going to be sitting in a corner staring at the floor on their smart phones.

They are there to work, and have their goals set in mind, therefore their mood is heavily exalted so people tend to look at each other, as humans do, and they could possibly glance your way from time to time. So if someone looks at you, glances over you, it's definitely not a sign of threat or your cue to run out and drive home. Everyone is there for his or her own personal reason and goals. In fact, we're all there for the same reason: to better ourselves. So plug your headphones in, play your favorite song and get into the workout without worrying if that man or woman over there is looking at you. If he is, well you better give them a good reason to stare! They are most likely admiring you for your efforts, if you are a beginner, or sometimes they just want to help you if they see you doing a movement wrong. You're better off getting support from someone at the gym for doing a wrong movement and are corrected on your form then pull a tendon, tear a muscle or break a bone. But most of the time it's just human nature to look around at others and see what others are doing. Some people are just nosey. If it's a blatant stare, you can always address it, or simply ignore it. No harm will come to you at the gym, I assure you that.

5. Stop worrying about the scale

The scale does not define you. Don't track everything on a day to day basis as our bodies are incredibly complex pieces of machinery where all kinds of crazy stuff happens all day and night therefore our weight fluctuates over the course of the day. Measuring every day will promote an unhealthy OCD behavior, where every little change will be scrutinized and blown out of proportion. Measure yourself once a week at the same time, after you wake up or before you eat your first meal. I choose Friday and Monday mornings to track measurements. The best ways to track are:

Taking a picture: Take a picture head on, to the side and a profile view. You might not like what you see and not want to look at it again nor show anyone but the picture holds you accountable and can be used in two months or three months for body transformation comparison through your transitional journey.

Take measurements: Buy a self-help tape measure and take a circumference measurement of these areas and write it down:

- Neck, shoulders, chest, bicep, waist, hips, thigh

Body fat percentage: No body fat percentage tracking is truly 100% accurate however ask at your local gym where you might be able to take one to give you a rough idea of how much fat you are holding

2 | FINDING YOUR FEET

You must hold yourself accountable. I am here to hold you accountable and help you reach your goals but ultimately it is up to you to complete your workouts and follow my instructions.

1. Remember that slow progress is progress

Never quit early. Think of your body like a plant. Watering your brand new plant may seem significant because it's new and green, and your sure it will last a while without maintenance and care, but day-by-day, it will start to willow and die. By watering it every day, it will grow to be strong and healthy. It may seem like slow progress but all those physiques you see out there and admire weren't built over night, they took years to build. Our bodies require tender loving care. Now water that plant, and get to work.

2. Visualize your future

Believe and achieve. Help your mind create a pattern for whatever it is you are visualizing. You can train your brain for something physical even though you're not actually doing anything physical. If you're in a negative state of mind, take a break to clear your mind. Try going outside for a few minutes, leave your desk, or put your phone down, and reflect on why you're in the position you're in then try again. The more detailed and realer your visualization, the more effective it will be. You can get your emotions involved as well. Feel what is like to go through that experience your visualizing. Visualization won't replace hard work but it will increase your chances of achieving your goals.

3. Set realistic goals

If you set yourself unrealistic goals you can end up feeling unmotivated and upset. Before you set your goal, be realistic, with where you are at now, if you are a complete beginner than start small with your goals and if you are in good shape then challenge yourself a bit more. For example: Don't keep telling yourself you're going to lose 2kg a week when it's not always realistic and sustainable. Sticking with the weight loss example, if you are a complete beginner then a good goal may be to lose 5kg in 3 months. If you're advanced a realistic goal may be 1kg per week. Set concise and measure goals each week or month and write them down before starting. Setting goals helps you stay on track. Use a diary or your smart phone as a way to stay consistent and track your days that you went to the gym and didn't, what you ate and did not, this way you have a cue to get back on track. Considering you probably glance at your phone at least twice every hour, use it as a means of helping you get to where you need to be.

4. Surround yourself with like-minded people

You can spend all your time on the Internet trolling celebrities or you can work hard at achieving your goals and reaching greatness. Surround yourself with people who uplift you and want the best for you. This is an excellent way to put your fitness goals on fast track. Birds of a feather flock together. I've seen a person's peer group be the difference between making successful fitness decisions and failing miserably. I've seen the same person lose weight and gain weight with just the change of surrounding influences. Get the people around you on board with your goals. Spend more time with those that will influence better decisions.

5. Cooking at home

The more you can cook at home, the more you will know exactly what is going into your system. When you eat out, you never know what the chef has put into your food to make it taste better. All they care about is that it taste good. Sugar, butter, and oil are often used in large quantities to flavor many dishes. That grilled chicken and vegetables you ordered isn't going to have the effect you're hoping for depending on the chef's recipe. Cooking at home is also cheaper and cost-effective.

6. Dissociating from bad habits or influences

Obesity runs in many families suggesting a belief that it's hereditary. Family habits are learned and observed by children at an early age however. They grow up with a certain lifestyle, and develop certain eating habits, and are usually fairly inactive, eventually creating the same image of their parents. Even a genetic predisposition can be overcome with healthy eating habits and a consistent exercise plan. Look at me, for example. My extended family tree has a history of diabetes, high blood pressure and obesity. My ancestry and cultural background also have a habit of overeating, as this is seen as a cultural significance; celebrating with large amounts of food, with very minimal controlled eating behaviors or patterns. Yet here I am. Studies have proven that obesity is more of a psychological problem that blooms into physical form as a symptom. Finding a healthy outlet to deal with emotional stress, anxiety, depression, and boredom instead of overeating would be an excellent start. The sooner the negative mentality is given up and responsibility is taken for one's body, the sooner change will begin.

3 | ARE YOU AN ECTOMORPH, MESOMORPH OR ENDOMORPH?

A lot of the time I hear people complain about their particular body type and compare themselves to others because of their particular shape. Sometimes I hear things like:

My body is not cut out for this.

I can never lose fat in my stomach area.

It's so much easier for other people to lose weight than me.

I wish I were born with abs.

What they are concerned about is called genetics. Genetics play a big role in how we look therefore impacting the results we get from exercising. A lot of people argue that genetics don't effect how our bodies react to exercise and fitness, I argue they do. For the most part genetics cannot be undone, obviously, however, there is a way to outsmart your genes by improving your exercise practices.

1. **Ectomorph – Lean and long build, flat chested, inward shoulders, small waist, lose fat quickly and struggle to put on weight**

My recommendation

Ditch the treadmill. You have a fast metabolism; an excessive amount of cardio is the last thing you need. Focus on compound exercises when strength training which means using more than one muscle group at a time to boost your testosterone levels, shock your body and stimulate growth. In saying that, leave the bicep curls and other singular muscle group exercises alone. Effective exercises for you include squats, overhead shoulder press and supersets where you jump between two exercises at once without taking a break or stopping. You also need to be eating at least every 2.5-3 hours, which is a lot, but this is required for growth. You should be having at least 112 grams of protein per day.

2. **Mesomorph – Naturally muscular build, high metabolism, responsive muscle cells, generally athletic body**

My recommendation

You generally put on quality mass quickly and have the ability to lose fat quickly too. You can get away with doing more cardio than necessary when you're weight lifting training often as your body's energy restores quickly and responds well to physical stimulus therefore not targeting your muscle as a source of energy. Honestly, you have it quite easy. You naturally are able to put on muscle mass without trying because your fat cells do not regenerate and build at a rapid pace. Your levels of testosterone are usually quite high making lean muscle mass easily attainable. Good for you!

3. **Endomorph – Wide, 'stocky' build, finds it hard to lost fat, high tendency to store body fat, slow metabolism, muscles not so defined**

My recommendation

Fasted cardio in the morning is your formula for fat loss. As soon as you wake up, hit the gym for a 30-minute treadmill session consisting of walking/jogging/running intervals. Walk for 30 seconds, jog for a minute, run for two minutes, etc. until your 20 minutes are up. Follow it up by 10 minutes of incline walking at your own pace and incline. The reason why I choose interval cardio training is because the more you consecutively "stop and start" during cardio, the more calories you burn. *Why?* Because it shocks your heart rate, causing your heart to pump out more blood throughout your body, burning more energy and more calories. However if you only stick to cardio and you are an Endomorph, you will lose fat but you will not gain much muscle, causing loose skin and a feeling of 'flatness' with no definition. You need to find a balance. You should still be lifting moderately heavy weight so I recommend cardio in the morning (before work/school/etc. if possible) and strength training at night. As someone who began as an Endomorph I understand the difficulty in losing fat, however combining cardiovascular activity with weight training twice a day, in what I refer to as a 'split-training program', paired with a nutritious, wholesome diet, which I explain in further detail soon, is the formula for success. Try this split workout for two weeks and witness the results.

4 | THE FORMULA FOR FAT LOSS

The Formula for fat loss is flexible eating paired with an understanding of how much to eat and when to eat. A firm understanding of the 3 macronutrients will assist you finding the right foods to eat to help with losing fat and building lean muscle. The general assumption is 'healthy eating' means eating broccoli, asparagus and brussel sprouts 24/7 but that's not the case. Learning about the various foods that are available to us creates room for us to enjoy various types of foods whilst still burning fat and building lean muscle. Once you learn what about what you like, find what your taste buds are attracted to, what your food requirements are and create a routine – one that works for you – the results will flow in.

Macronutrient breakdown

1. **Protein** essential for muscle repair, rebuilding and putting on muscle mass
    - **Harder training days:** At least 1180 calories of protein per day
    - **Low training days:** At least 1150 calories of protein per day

2. **Carbohydrates** needed to fuel workouts, protein synthesis, muscle growth, and sugar replenishment (healthy sugars)
    - **Harder training days:** At least 1300 calories of carbs per day
    - **Low training days:** At least 1000 calories of carbs per day

3. **Healthy fats** needed for hormone development and energy levels
    - **Harder training days:** At least 800 calories of fats per day
    - **Low training days:** At least 700 calories of fats per day

✓ **High training day average calories**: Around 3300 calories per day

✓ **Low training day average calories**: Around 2900 calories per day

The calories mentioned above are required for putting on large amounts of muscle mass and contribute to fat loss also. However, when multiplied by the days in the week, this is a very large amount of calories for a beginner to process and consume in just one week, without a doubt, especially one who is so used to eating only once or twice a day! **I have only included the calories above as an idea for you to understand the calories that you would need to be consuming if you want to put on a lot of muscle mass.** Therefore I advise you to go slow and pace yourself carefully. Don't let the numbers scare you away. There is no rush. There are other ways of getting to where you need to be. That being said, as I mentioned at the beginning, monitoring your diet through flexible dieting is one of the main sources of fat loss. So you don't have actually count your calories! As long as you are consuming one of the 3 macronutrients mentioned above on a regular basis in every meal you are having; then you are 95% of the way there.

Proteins

This macro is what we all think of when it comes to building muscle. It is responsible for muscle repair that's been broken down from hard resistance training or excessive cardio and it is responsible for keeping new muscle mass on whilst burning fat. So if you are at a state right now where you feel you have plateaued in your training, here are some **quality protein sources** to consider:

- Lean chicken, beef, lamb, turkey, pork
- Fresh fish, canned fish
- Deli meat (turkey and ham)
    - – Consider the amount you consume as this is can be processed depending on place of purchase. Always ask how it's prepared.
- Beef broth
- Tendon meat from beef, chicken, lamb, pork
- Dairy (milk, cheese, yogurt)
- Egg whites

Carbohydrates

Without carbs, there is no growth. Carbs are necessary for performance and improved body composition (shaping of your body). When you rid your body of carbs, your body starts to break down the protein you've eaten as well as your muscles to use as sugar (glucose). The human brain runs on glucose. So technically what your brain needs to function, you're banning it's life source, and in turn causing it to reach for whatever else it can to function. That is how you lose muscle mass and that is how you feel flat/slim/drained.

Carbs store in your muscles and are the primary fuel source for your high-intensity activities. Some **quality carbohydrate sources** to consider:

- Potatoes (all varieties, namely sweet potato)
- Rice (brown)
- Pasta
- Fruit
- Fresh fruit juice (no concentrated or supermarket juice)
- All vegetables
- Bread (anything but white)
- Grains

Fats

Good fats are essential nutrients to absorb the disappearing vitamins in our blood stream. Some vitamins go into our bodies but unfortunately we don't get the use out of them because they're absorbed in our blood for other uses around the body, uses the body finds more important. (Remember our bodies aren't designed to look the way we expect them to. We have to tailor our lifestyles to that requisite.) Fat is the backup source behind carbs for energy. A diet too low in fat can slow down hormone production be it testosterone or estrogen. Quality fat sources include:

- Coconut oil (I highly recommend sautéing your chicken with this one day)
- Palm oil
- Olive oil (extra virgin)
- Beef, lamb (grass-fed)
- Avocado
- Egg yolks (if you have high cholesterol avoid this)
- Dark chocolate (reasonable amounts!)
- Nuts (almond, brazil nuts, macadamia nuts)

Pricing

In general living a healthy lifestyle with a flexible diet will be more expensive than eating one meal a day for the whole week or having potato chips for dinner, some items are more expensive than others, but it's an investment into your health and a price you have to be willing to pay. You can choose to eat McDonalds six nights a week or choose to spend your money on alcohol every weekend, but the decision remains with you as does your future and goals. You also have to shop around. Particularly with organic foods, which is my personal preference as non-organic labels or brands tend to use herbicides which is damaging to our insides. At the end of the day it comes down to affordability and what you can manage. As long as you're trying, doing your best and working towards building a healthier lifestyle, setting things into place then that's what matters. If you can afford to buy organic then do so, as I recommend this.

Flexible eating

'Clean eating' is an aggressive over-used term that clouds a lot of people's judgment and thought process when it comes to eating, scaring them away from all the confusion of what's good and what's bad. A flexible diet allows for range and options. 80% of the times you must make sure you eat a variety of wholesome foods to receive your vitamin, mineral, and energy requirements and stimulate muscle growth and fat loss, and 20% of the time, you can actually enjoy whatever you like. However 20% should not be a great deal. Listen to your body, feel the change, what's working and what's not, start cooking at home, trial and error how your body reacts to this change in your eating and you will get the hang of it. If you feel you are not moving then your 20% needs to be reduced to 5% or 10% and your 80% needs to be upped to at least 90% and you must commit.

Foods to consider

- All fruits and vegetables
    - Apples, bananas, watermelon, mango, oranges
    - Broccoli
    - Cauliflower
    - Onion
    - Green beans
    - Asparagus
    - Spinach
    - Kale
    - Garlic
    - Radishes
    - Brussel sprouts
    - Tomatoes
    - Fennel
    - Cabbage
    - Lemon/Limes
    - Beets
- Animal products for your source of protein (unless vegan or vegetarian) i.e. muscle and organ meat, dairy products also
    - See proteins mentioned above
- Grains, potatoes, rice
    - Sweet potato/Yams
    - Oats
    - Muesli
    - Lentils
    - Basmati rice
    - Brown rice
    - Wild rice
    - Gluten free pasta
    - Gluten free bread slice (1 slice a day)

        - Preferably Ezekiel, Rye or Multigrain
- Saturated and unsaturated oils i.e. coconut, olive, palm oils
- Healthy fats
    - Almonds (15 a day only)
    - Macadamia nuts (4)
    - Brazil nuts (3)
    - 1 tablespoon of almond butter
    - 1 tablespoon of peanut butter

Foods to avoid

- Anything packaged with a long shelf life i.e. cookies, cakes, pastries, etc.
- Readily available frying oil i.e. mostly hydrogenated oils
- Deep fried foods
- Anything you would get at a fast food restaurant
- Soft drinks/soda
- Overly processed sweet, candy and confectionary
- Artificial sweeteners
    - A Diet Coke or Coke Zero is not a supplement for a drink. *"But it has zero sugar!"* The taste of something sweet elicits an insulin spike. Basically it signals your body to eat, when it actually doesn't need food at all disrupting your feeling of being 'full'.

Craving control options

- 1 peach = 37 calories
- ½ grapefruit = 37 calories
- 1 cup sliced strawberries = 50 calories

1 cup watermelon pieces = 51 calories

- 1 cup papaya pieces = 54 calories
- ¾ apricot halves = 55 calories
- 1 cup cantaloupe cubes = 56 calories
- 1 orange = 60 calories
- Herbal teas (as many as you like)
- 2 large celery stalks = 13 calories
- 2 cups shredded romaine lettuce = 18 calories
- ½ cucumber = 20 calories
- 1 medium tomato = 25 calories
- 1/3 cup sugar snap peas = 30 calories
- 1 carrot = 30 calories
- 1 cup jicama sticks = 45 calories
- 12 almonds = 84 calories

Portion control

One of the biggest contributors to fat gain is portion size being completely off.

You don't need to count calories to get the right portions for your goals. Instead, just use your hand to measure. This keeps meal times simple and easy. Now that we have reached the end of this chapter, you should have learned more information about specific foods and nutrients.

Portion control using your hands:

- A portion of protein = 1 palm
- A portion of vegetables = 1 fist
- A portion of carbs = 1 cupped hand
- A portion of fats = 1 thumb

Start planning your meals with this basic template that's customized for you. You can always individualize further as you go along.

5 | CONSISTENCY

Stop constantly rewarding yourself with unhealthy food after a good streak.

I've been so good all week long, so I'm going to have a pizza.

I'm going to drink a whole bottle of wine because it's movie night!

It's my friend's birthday so we're celebrating by getting wasted this weekend! I'll burn it off when I get back to the gym on Monday.

Basically, let's undo everything that you just spent all week working hard for. You spend days working your butt off during the week, trying to look good for yourself, that date you have next Friday night, your summer body, etc. Yet you're so close to your goals and losing all that fat that you have been wanting to lose for so long… But you decide to unnecessarily treat yourself to some take away foods or a few shots at the club. The next day you will wake up to find you've put on weight with severe bloating and an upset tummy. Consistency is key. Your body flushes out all the bad toxins from your blood stream throughout the week as you eat healthy and train harder and harder each day that when the day comes and you decide to 'cheat', your body automatically goes into panic mode and starts reaching for the fat storage for energy and protection. In addition, after 6 days of perfection, you find you have lost a couple of pounds on the scale and decide to "take a break". The next day you have completely yo-yoed back into the same place you were at the beginning of the week and sometimes even further behind.

Success happens when you spend months being perfectly on point, developing new habits and restructuring your body, boosting your metabolic rate, and making bad foods a foreign entity that the body can't remember and is not used to processing. It seems unrealistic and impossible but it's not. I did it. Why can't you? Only at that point, once you have achieved a level of consistency, dedication and commitment can you get away with that type of celebration. You will know when. What is interesting though, is the people who get to that point, have actually lost all desire to celebrate in that way because their body is no longer interested or craving those things anymore. You can't think of it as a sacrifice. If you do, you will be miserable. You have to think of it as developing a new mindset and a new lifestyle if you want to be successfully consistent long term and achieve your goals.

By being consistent with your training, you are elevating your metabolic rate allowing your body to burn calories well after you have stopped training. Any activity is better than no activity – if there are days where you think you have no time to workout well, you are lying to yourself. Time can always be made for moving around and being somewhat active.

6 | WHEN SHOULD I EAT?

You must stick to an eating schedule that suits your lifestyle.

Eating 6 to 8 small meals per day to make your metabolism faster is a myth. If you eat all your necessary calories that you need to eat for the day in 1 meal or space them out, the results will be the same. Obviously we want to space them out so you do not starve.

'Time restricted feeding' is a better way of viewing timing. It is not a specific way of telling when you should time each meal, but it tells you a feeding period of when you can eat. This is also referred to as 'intermittent fasting'. Before you freak out by the name – I won't let you starve.

The time period for the best results varies anywhere from a 12 hour eating period and an 8 hour eating period. The period starts and finishes when you first ingest something that isn't water including your first cup of coffee for the day – whatever gets your body going in the morning. Your eating clock starts the moment you eat something that isn't water. Holding off on the first bite or sip allows you to start feeding later in the day.

Implementing time restricted feeding

You want to end your feeding period 2-3 hours before you go to bed. So if you sleep at 10pm then your last meal should be at 7 to 8pm. It is best to halt our eating before 7pm so that our body can properly digest our food and soak in all the nutrients because if we fall asleep for 7 to 8 hours where our body enters a sleeping mode and fasting state, then nothing happens but rest – which is fantastic for your health but your body doesn't effectively digest all the nutrients needed for muscle growth after this time.

So let's use 7pm as the end of our feeding period for example. I am also only using 3 meals as an example but you are welcome to 4, 5 or even 6 depending on portions.

A 12-hour fast/12-hour feeding period would look like:

- 7am = Meal 1
- 12pm = Meal 2
- 5pm = Meal 3
- 7pm = Snack

A 16-hour fast/8-hour eating period would look like:

- 11am = Meal 1
- 2pm = Meal 2
- 5pm = Meal 3
- 7pm = Snack

Remember these are just examples and you can change the meal times within the feeding period to better suit you as long as you stick to the feeding period.

7 | WORST SUBSTANCE FOR YOUR BODY

Alcohol is the worst thing you can put in your body.

Firstly, let's talk about Insulin. Insulin is a hormone in the pancreas that allows for fat storage because it spikes your sugar levels. Although we all have it in our body we need to do our best to avoid consuming foods that trigger a large amount of insulin. We trigger Insulin by consuming foods high in sugar. Alcohol triggers insulin for up to 36 hours in your body because of the amount of sugar in it meaning your body has 36 hours to store as much fat as it can and do whatever it likes with it.

I'll drink water to flush it out.

I'll eat something really greasy and full of carbs to soak it all up.

That's incorrect. That won't work. No matter what you eat after alcohol in an attempt to 'soak' it up, it has already secured a spot in your bloodstream and is now playing catch-ups with your fat cells. Your body has 36 hours to do whatever it wants with alcohol and no matter what you eat afterwards, it's floating around in your bloodstream and is being stored in your body as fat. So, you're screwed. Just kidding. Not really. Start cutting alcohol out of your diet and watch those abs start to appear under the layer of fat that the alcohol is helping to form.

Alcohol lowers testosterone levels too. Testosterone is the male sex hormone that helps build muscle and lowers fat levels. In fact, alcohol does the opposite effect of what testosterone should do. It increases estrogen levels, which causes water retention, bloating and more fat storage. Dehydration is another side effect of alcohol. You might wonder why your mouth gets so dry after a night out, well that's because your body is made up of 60% water. Alcohol sucks the water and nutrients out of your body, causing dehydration, bad skin, breath, yellow teeth, bloating, etc. For every alcoholic drink you have, you're wasting 36 hours of your life reducing your chances of fat loss and removing vitamins from your body needed for growth and progression.

8 | SUPERFOODS

Some of the best foods out there that I like to consider Superfoods, which aid in fat loss and have super health benefits.

Water based

Celery

The wonders of food are made evident through celery. This literally helps you lose fat. You can consume celery and know you're burning fat. It has the highest negative calorie content of any food because the digestion of the green stalk burns 25 calories. It contains 6 calories for every 8-inch of a stalk, giving it a 19 calorie deficit to the body. A cup of celery a day, helps the fat go away. *Best served as a snack wherever whenever. Add some lemon and you're good to go!*

Water

You should be consuming at least 1 liter of water a day. It shocks me when people don't drink any water. I drink on average 2-3 litres water a day. Yes, I do pee a lot. But the benefits I reap are incredible including maximum physical performance, treatment of headaches, constipation, brain function, and the physical benefits such as clear skin, silky hair, healthier teeth, no bad breathe, and the list goes on! *Start making it an effort to carry a bottle of water everywhere you go. If I can carry a 3-litre bottle everywhere I go then you can carry a 600ml bottle.*

Chili and spices

Cayenne pepper

The hotness of the food stimulates the hypothalamus in our body to reset the body's fat temperature causing the body to burn off excess fat and keeps the body from storing fat alongside muscular tissues which is the stubborn fat deep inside that makes us feel all soft and mushy. *Easily used to season foods, particularly main meals containing proteins or red meats.*

Cinnamon extract

This is not the same as cinnamon sugar or cinnamon oil. It helps with blood glucose levels; supports healthy cholesterol levels, regulates stable blood pressure, and improves body composition. It's a must for anyone prone to type II Diabetes. It can be found at your local chemist or pharmacy. *Consume alongside a meal containing a portion of protein.*

Breakfast foods or snack foods

Acai

A powerful food that stimulates your metabolism and calorie consumption rate and lowers your blood pressure and cholesterol. Found in Brazil, it contains more antioxidants than any other food in the world. Antioxidants keep your cells alive, therefore Acai helps build our immune system preventing cancer, breathing problems, heart conditions, diseases, etc. and combating our fat cells. *I like to have my acai in the morning with rolled oats and almond milk.*

Fruits and vegetables

Broccoli

One of the healthiest foods you can consume is Broccoli. Contains enzymes and high fiber content that fights colon cancer, tumors and other forms of cancer such as breast cancer in women. It also helps keep you regular and stimulates muscle growth. There are only 34 calories in 100 grams of broccoli. *I like to have my broccoli steamed with lemon and pepper next to my protein of choice.*

Apples

Apples aid in digestion and provide as much dietary fiber as a bowl of bran cereal. Due to being so high in fiber apples make you feel fuller for longer periods of time therefore adding it to your diet intake can be super beneficial when you have cravings especially night cravings. Being so high in dietary fiber, they help with fat loss. No more than two apples a day as they do contain sugar. *I enjoy my apples throughout the day, when I am on the go I make sure I have a few green apples sliced and diced in a container helping to keep me regular also.*

Carrots

Have you ever struggled with sexual dysfunction? Trim the skin off 4 carrots; pour about 250ml of water into your blender and blend. Then drink. Carrots help with low sex drive amongst many other things such as eyesight, constipation and dandruff. They also aid in fat loss being soluble meaning their nutrients absorb well into our bloodstream. *Enjoyed best as a juice or sliced with a bit of lemon squeezed on top.*

Spinach

Have you seen Popeye? Spinach is a super food with high levels of iron that helps our muscles store oxygen looking fuller and healthier. Spinach is exceptional for people with anemia. Although when cooked or steamed, because of its oxalic acid content, the iron can be reduced therefore by adding red meats next to your spinach it helps increase our body's chance of absorbing all of the iron. The nutrients latch onto the red meat and don't get washed away when absorbed in the body giving us muscles! *I enjoy my spinach steamed, sometimes raw but washed well, next to my lean mince turkey or 99% fat free lean red meat of choice, or even my chicken! A dash of pepper goes a long way.*

Onions

Onions contain antioxidants, helping keep your insides nice and refreshed. Although they might give you bad breath occasionally, they are working hard to keep your skin clear and hair soft. Raw onion is known to lower the production of bad cholesterol and keep your heart healthy. An entire onion makes up more than one cup of water! *A few slices of onion in every meal lightly sautéed or raw if you're brave enough will 100% keep your skin feeling amazing.*

Beets

A lot of processed meats found in takeaway foods cause cancer in the stomach. If you eat a lot of processed food, start cleaning up your habits by eating beets. The red color of the beet contains an active enzyme that gets the liver working to break down and fights cancerous cells. Beets also flush water through the system to get rid of any water retention if you're feeling bloated. *Best served in a salad with rocket, pumpkin and walnuts.*

Garlic

Garlic has the ability to burn fat by operating in a similar way to cayenne pepper. Through its active ingredients, it stimulates the body's temperature and hypothalamus causing the body to burn fat. *Easily used alongside foods containing proteins, particularly main meals such as lunch or dinner, or even salads.*

Ginger

Ginger increases production of lactic acid in our body, which increases the body's rate at which it burns fat. Lactic acid stimulates growth hormones, which increase the breakdown of fat cells. *Easily used alongside foods containing proteins, particularly main meals such as lunch or dinner, or even salads.*

9 | SUPPLEMENTS

Please be aware of purchasing supplements online. I strongly recommend buying all supplements face to face unless from a reputable online website or brand

Vitamin supplements

Magnesium

- For someone with a poor diet who lacks magnesium rich foods such as fish, nuts beans, vegetables, I would recommend taking it in the form of a standard dose of 200mg
- It can cause an upset tummy if you don't take it with food and water
- I also don't recommend getting used to taking it in the form of a supplement out of a bottle, meaning you should start to get used to incorporating fish and vegetables in your diet
- Helps with bone health and joint recovery after workouts

Vitamin D

- Standard 50-70mcg dosage with food high in fat, either year round or in the colder, darker months where you're not exposed to vitamin D from the sun
- Anything more than 75mcg should only be considered if you have a severe deficiency of vitamin D (blood test screening will show this)

Zinc

- Requirements vary depending on if you sweat much during your workouts or perform at a high level and if you consume enough read meat, if you do both you might not need this supplement at all but I would still limit myself to 10-20mg/day

Supplements to support muscle building

Whey protein (1 scoop)

- Prevent muscle breakdown
- Your body is most likely to feed off your muscle at night time, due to the long period that it goes without food
- Whey protein is more important after a hard weight training workout because the body absorbs it quickly, it will deliver the essential proteins within the hour.
- I usually have a shake in the morning for breakfast to break the fast, and a shake after my workout

BCAAs (1 scoop)

- Commonly talked about but the combination of the three amino acids they contain make up 1/3 of our skeletal muscle in the human body
- Protein synthesis support
- I drink them either throughout the day, or if I don't have enough time because I'm struggling to balance everything in the day, I drink them during my workout

Creatine monohydrate (1 scoop)

- 1-2 hours before exercise, take
- Draws water in the muscle cells creating size and strength
- Creates potential for more muscular endurance, faster recovery and lean muscle mass
- Must replenish your body with lots of water for this to work so drink up because your body relies on water when creatine is ingested

L-Citrulline (10g malate)

- Half an hour before exercise to help with high energy levels, increased blood flow and maximum performance while working out

NO2 (nitric oxide)

- Increases blood flow and oxygen throughout the body to our muscles to help keep us pumped without fatigue through our workouts and then some afterwards

Supplements to support with fat loss

OxyShred (1 scoop)

- 30 minutes before exercise

- A fat burner that helps with fat breakdown in your body, can be used as a pre workout due to high amounts of sugar

Lipo 6

- Caffeine in a controlled intake is an excellent fat burning substance
- Lipo 6 is a product combining caffeine other fat burning components compacted in a liquid gel capsule

Highly recommended supplements to keep weight off

Omega-6 fatty acids help burn fat and are good for preventing weight gain after you've lost weight. They also help to control appetite. So if you're on a strictly weight loss journey and want to keep the weight off, I highly recommend these. These can be found in your local supplement store, chemist or pharmacy.

GLA (gamma linolenic acid) or GLA-90

- GLA is a good appetite suppressant to help you feel full and eat less if you're going through a weight loss journey with sound understanding of what you're meant to be eating and not.
- GLA also helps the skin maintain tone and stay moisturized so it doesn't sag after or during weight loss.

CLA or CLA-1000

- CLA is burns stubborn fat, the kind hiding in between muscles and organs, and especially belly fat.
- Research published in the International Journal of Obesity (August 2001) found that a group of overweight

men taking CLA lost mostly belly fat and reduced their waistlines by 1 inch without making any diet or lifestyle changes.

- While CLA helps burn fat, it helps gain lean muscle at the same time.
- A yearlong research study performed by the Scandinavian Clinical Research Group in 2007 found that overweight people lost 9% of their body fat and increased their lean muscle mass by 2% just by taking CLA with no changes in their diet or lifestyle.
- A University of Wisconsin-Madison study in 2008 concluded that CLA helped to prevent weight gain in people who previously lost weight.

10 | STARVING YOURSELF

If you or anyone you know is suffering from an eating disorder and believe it is uncontainable, and are in need of urgent help, I warmly recommend seeking professional help through an organization or foundation that represents all people affected by eating disorders and/or negative body image or calling a 24/7 eating disorder treatment hotline.

Starving yourself, or eating one meal a day, causes your metabolism to suffer. It doesn't make you burn fat. It makes you gain weight, or causes you too plateau, deplete, feel weak, flat, etc. If you go too far below your maintenance calories per day – calories you need to survive on for the day and do regular human activities – your body goes into starvation mode. When you starve, you shed any muscle you had and your body stores calories as fat for a future energy source. Meaning as soon as you start eating again your body stores it as fat for precaution. Not eating enough wholesome foods that support fat loss also lowers the amount of calories you burn. Less supportive meals equals less body fat burned. This can lead to thyroid issues, which I suffered from for many years because I starved myself in my teenage years.

The problem is the minute you go off any super strict diet that isn't flexible enough for your needs, the weight is going to come piling on. Keeping a super strict diet for long term will also be difficult because you are not enjoying what you're eating therefore making you miserable and welcoming a whole wave of other issues you would have to face.

The truth is people who have managed to stay slim all their lives without exercise are technically still holding a lot of fat. When you don't feed your body, it stores everything you do feed it. Your body holds onto every bad calorie even when you're not eating. What better way to hold onto it, then to store it in a fat cell, where it can only be used as a source of energy when needed at a later time. *Making sense?* You must incorporate flexible dieting that allows you to eat 80% healthy and 20% enjoy foods you normally would, to both nourish your body, achieve your fitness goals and also to stay sane. You don't want to turn yourself off food, as complications can be long term.

Overcoming my eating disorder

I suffered from bulimia in my early teens. My eating disorder fluctuated from bulimia to anorexia. It was a dark time for me. I wasn't sure whether I wanted to starve myself or over-indulge, force it out and then repeat. It was just an endless loop of nowhere. I had obsessive bingeing episodes and ate nothing on some days, and other days I would eat everything, purge (vomit it out), and repeat. Stereotypes about dieting and weight can lead medical health professionals to overlook or mischaracterize important physical, emotional and social signs and symptoms of eating disorders.

If we look at an eating disorder in a methodical approach, it can be somewhat comforting to realize that there is light at the end of the tunnel; every step just takes time and proactivity.

The steps I followed

1. At some point during your episode, you will hit what you feel is your lowest point. You must realize you have a disorder and *want* to get help. Reading recovery stories online did help me. Stories and experiences helped me to believe that if other people made it out then I would too. If all possibilities feel inevitable prior to understanding the need for help, please reach out to a local organization that assists with eating disorders. There is always someone waiting to listen and wanting to help.
2. The second step would be to rid yourself of anything that triggers your disorder that either make you feel worse or stimulate comparisons, including photos, social media, networking, toxic friends or people in your life, etc., even your phone.
3. Transparency, although hard to face, is the third step to recovery; so opening up to a loved one helps for example. Sometimes this could be a friend, doctor or counselor, if you believe your family won't understand. Some people are closer with their friends then they are family, or vice versa. I recommend always opening up to at least one family member. They are your family and will always try to understand what you're going through.
4. Joining a recovery community, organization or foundation is the next step to your recovery. There are others out there going through what you are going through. You are never alone. The feelings you are feeling, other people have felt and overcame. Therefore so can you. You can do it together. Humans were not created to be alone.

5. Following a structured eating program is the next step. You will begin noticing a dramatic reduction in your symptoms with the help of medical professionals as well as your counselor or support system. Recovery won't be easy. I had relapses, mood swings, and anxiety attacks, and bloating and weight fluctuations but a willingness to get better is what got me through.
6. Staying close with your support system and avoiding triggers begins to clear the fog. Old parts of your personality will return. You become less anxious and more centered. Vision becomes clearer and the light at the end of the tunnel is right there in front of you. You are yourself again.

11 | SURGERY

The purpose of this chapter is to inform and educate readers on differentiating between natural and surgical methods of weight loss to prevent comparisons and understand the difference between natural methods and surgical.

It is important to note that you never know what surgery(s) someone has undergone, unless you have the knowledge and understanding in the field of fitness, beauty, cosmetics, etc., therefore it is important to be aware of this and to never compare yourself because for an everyday person, they can believe the works of surgery are attainable naturally. You just don't know the circumstance of someone else so you will do well to not compare your hard work to that of other's otherwise it can result in self-defeat. Everyone's journey is different and I cannot emphasize this enough. Comparisons are unhealthy, particularly when people who have had surgery claim to be natural, misleading you. Everyone is entitled to do whatever they like with their bodies therefore I strongly urge you to focus only on yourself and your path and not that of others who have thousands of dollars disposable at their hands to alter their appearance however they see fit. You can do the same safely and naturally.

There are two types of surgeries:

1. **Cosmetic procedures to enhance or alter your appearance**
    a. Costs anywhere between $8000.00 to $20,000 depending on areas of the body that are enhanced or altered
    b. Usually undergone in a clinic, sometimes private clinics or clinics that don't provide overnight care
    c. Designed to re-shape and contour your body **not help with fat loss**
    d. Fat can be put back on with bad eating habits or poor exercise
    e. Anyone can undergo this procedure as long as you have the money
    f. Most common: Injections, implants, liposuction or the most common: fat transfer where fat is removed and deposited in other areas of the body for a larger appearance

2. **Weight loss procedures to help you burn fat**
    a. Costs anywhere between $10,000 to $18,000
    b. Usually undergone in a hospital with a registered doctor or bariatric
    c. Usually reduces the size of your stomach, stomach lining and appetite
    d. 3 most common: Gastric sleeve, bypass or lap-band
    e. You have to be considered obese and at adverse or life-threatening risk and deteriorating health to have permission to undergo this procedure

How to differentiate natural musculature from cosmetic surgery

The thighs, hamstrings and calves should always match the entire musculature of the lower body. Consistency where the butt meets the hamstring should be evident and where it is not we can assume surgery has impacted the area. There is no possible way to build your butt without building the rest of your lower body with it. There is a fast growing population undergoing fat transfer procedures to alter the size of their waists and butt by transferring visceral fat to other parts of their bodies to appear fuller, bigger, wider or thicker. By avoiding cosmetic procedures, you can avoid health complications, debt, bodily scarring, future impediments, and your portions not complementing. The biggest reward is the fulfillment of knowing you did it all on your own. You are stronger than you know.

12 | STEROIDS

Adverse side effects and health complications do exist in the health and fitness industry where steroids are used. Steroids are used as performance enhancers to help you grow in size, put on fast muscle and lose fat quickly. They can be used in a relatively safe manner if you know what you are doing and/or you are under the supervision of a doctor or a professional bodybuilding mentor but this does not make side effects any less preventable. In 2017 5 prominent bodybuilders passed away from excessive steroid use, heart or liver complications.

Steroids require strict commitment and dedication. They do not get you the results you want within two months by simply injecting them into your body. If you do not maintain a special regime for a consistent period of time for up to 12 or more weeks and accompany the lifestyle required for it you do not see results. Meaning, having a full time job can be very hard when balancing your commitment to steroids and working out 2 to 3 times a day. Professionals in the fitness industry who have had access to steroids for years usually distribute steroids, otherwise doctors are able to also but only medicinally. They are quite costly to purchase and to maintain, averaging about $90-$120 per bottle in some countries. A bodybuilder taking steroids can spend up to $3000.00 on just 12 to 16 weeks worth of steroids. In the late 2000s production of steroids began being strongly monitored and they are now considered illegal in many countries today.

How to tell if someone is on steroids or not

1. Sudden unexpected transformation

In just a month or two, they have become twice their regular size with large amounts of vascularity and thick prominent veins. They have a very 'dry', lean or shredded appearance with protruding muscles clearly visible after a small period of time (six to eight weeks) Steroids offer quick and impressive results by boosting testosterone levels and stimulating muscle growth. Large transformations definitely occur naturally but take a longer time (usually four to six months) with a strict workout and diet regime.

2. Gynecomastia (male breasts)

Observed in many young men at a young age (I had this growing up), when it is visible in grown men with muscular physiques and a great amount of muscle, we can conclude that steroids are involved. Caused by an excess intake of testosterone, which converts, to estrogen (female sex hormone), leading to high amounts of the female hormone creating breast tissue and a white ring around the nipples.

3. Stretch marks

Stretch marks are very common in weight loss and muscle growth and effect men and women alike. Obviously anyone can get stretch marks and it doesn't necessarily mean they are on steroids but how we can tell is when men rapidly grow and expand at a greater than normal capacity and speed, particularly the shoulder, biceps and chest area where the muscles connect; deep blue/purple stretch marks begin to sprout and we can assume it is the cause of steroids.

4. 'GH gut' or Growth Hormone gut

Some bodybuilders who enter popular bodybuilding contests use a hormone called Growth Hormone, which stimulates every part of your body to grow even your organs and your skull. Their stomachs usually end up protruding but their abs still clearly defined. Growth Hormones stimulate organ growth, which is impossible naturally. By enlarging your organs, it also enlarges the fat in the lining of your stomach therefore the stomach will inevitably poke out.

5. Back acne and grainy skin

Steroids make your skin very acne prone because a lot of steroids are oil-based liquids, which trigger the oil glands to become super active, hence causing parts of your body to break out. Acne can be found on the back, face, chest and butt when using steroids. Acne happens to anyone of course, but if a certain part of a man's body who is muscular and large in size has cystic acne on particularly large muscular areas, it can be concluded as steroids. Another skin condition steroids can cause is commonly known as 'grainy skin'. It's self-explanatory, as the skin looks grainy and sand-like sprouting small brown blemishes.

Conclusion

As stated in my *'Surgery'* chapter, unless you have sound judgment of the fitness industry it is crucial to never compare yourself to that of a bodybuilder who has been in the game for over 15 years and has sacrificed a 'normal' lifestyle to dedicate their life to the art of bodybuilding involving consistent steroid use by choice. If you are a person with a full time job and other life commitments, you can start to believe the work of steroids is attainable naturally, which they are not, which is the purpose of steroids, to obtain a physique that can't be naturally obtained and achieve optimum physical performance and strength faster, thus feeling defeated because what you have tried isn't working on you and all these thoughts start to cloud your judgment about how you feel about yourself and the gym and before you know it you're going home defeated! Stop worrying about what others are doing! Everyone's journey is different and I cannot emphasize this enough. Comparisons are unhealthy, particularly when enhancements are involved. Focus on yourself.

13 | THE TRUTH ABOUT CARDIO

Allow me to explain the common misconception that doing vigorous hours of cardio a day or week will help you lose all the fat you are holding in your body. Sure, hours of cardio will definitely assist you in reducing fat but it's not the solution to all your fat problems especially loose skin and your cravings afterwards. If you want to tighten your skin, grow your muscles, make sure your body goes after the right foods and your mind doesn't switch to unhealthy foods straight after a cardio session, you need a good balance of cardio and strength training.

Doing an endless amount of steady cardio will hinder your progress. Recommended amount of cardio to promote cardiovascular conditioning (positive heart rate) and fat burning is generally three days a week – on weight-lifting days or after weight lifting sessions. So by splitting up your training you promote growth and strength.

The 2 times in the day when cardio is most effective when wanting to lose fat

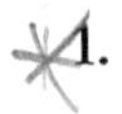

1. In the morning before breakfast – known as 'fasted cardio'
    - When you first wake up is one of the most effective times to do cardio
    - Your body has been without food for hours and is ready to access the emergency storage for energy, also known as the fat cells

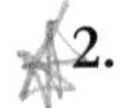

2. After a long workout/weight lifting session
    - All your energy levels are drained

Why? Because your body has been fasting during these periods with no food meaning and all the energy levels in your muscles are low. Let me explain. Fat burning activates only when the body has no more supplies of energy to use after all the main supplies of energy have been used. Let me explain a bit more. The hours of cardio you are doing are using the first sources on command: the food in your stomach and the energy in your muscles. Those are two sources that cardio drains first. ***Only then*** after these two sources are completely drained, the body starts drawing at the fat. Make sense? *Why does the body do this?* Well because your body wants to hold on to fat! So it will do everything to draw on other things before it does fat! *What do we need to do in this case?* Let's read on!

How much cardio should I do?

We must enter the 'burning fat zone' and stay in it. Your body is going to go into survival mode if you exceed the burning fat zone limit. Which means it's going to hold onto the fat, it's number one source of energy, and burn the muscle instead. This is why so many people feel 'flat' after cardio! *You mean all those miles I've been running; I've just been burning the muscle that I've worked so hard for?* Yes! It's important not to exceed 20 to 30 minutes of cardio at a time, if your goal is fat loss. The burning zone reaches around the 15-minute mark and onwards when doing high intensity cardio. When the heart rate of the body is elevated for long periods of time, there's a good chance your body will go back into survival mode and hold onto the fat. Don't get me wrong; you will still lose fat doing higher intensity cardio for long periods of time but it just won't be successfully targeting the fat like it could.

Must-do cardio exercises

Approaching cardio equipment can be daunting because you're unsure of what to do or what they do for you. I like to select cardio machines that target fat loss but also help me keep my muscle mass on without burning too much of it off. If you tend to feel 'flat' or 'drained' or – *I hate using this word* – 'scrawny, after cardio, therefore you must avoid doing cardio that makes you feel this way. To prevent this sensation and not feel depleted, you must do cardio exercises that use your muscles as well as your heart rate. Exercises that mainly use your heart rate are good for things like building stamina, breath control, and losing fat but not necessarily building muscle. Adding in resistance (pressure) to your cardio helps build muscle.

You can choose to these exercises together or do them separately, obviously if you do both; the better results you will see and the bigger your butt will get. This is not my butt workout that can be found at the very end of *The Formula* but these are definitely necessary additions to helping your butt grow bigger in between leg day or during leg day. Again it all depends on your scheduling, the time you have on your hands, and how much you wish to commit to your health, muscle building and fat loss.

1. **Stair master**

For a muscle-building workout, I like to do short bursts on the Stairmaster for 1-3 minutes with a high intensity level implemented, followed by 20 squats off the machine for a total of 15 minutes, two times a week. The highest level for the Stairmaster range between levels 15 to 20. You need at least level 15 to get the results you want. You will find as you increase the level, the trick becomes staying up on the machine, as you will notice your feet falling, or trembling to the ground. You should be completely out of breath after a few minutes on the machine. Complete 1-3 minutes, jump off and perform 20 body squats in the air, jump back on and complete another 3 minutes and continue until you've reached your 15th minute. Good luck walking the next few days.

2. **Incline treadmill walking**

This is as an alternative to your Stairmaster, if you don't have it at your gym or if you have decided you want to do fasted cardio in the morning, that I explained above as being crucially beneficial to fat loss. Incline walking can help you burn fat super quickly while tightening your muscles in your butt and toning it. A steady incline walk can build strength in your glutes much better than walking, sprinting, jogging or running can. By walking uphill you are using the muscles in your butt and hamstrings that make your butt grow thicker and wider. Adjust your incline (uphill slope) on a level between 5.0 to 8.0 and walk on a steady pace between 5.5 to 6.0 for a total of 15 minutes.

Determining your maximum heart rate

The formula to determine this is: 220 – Your age

- Example: If you are 28
- 220-28 = 192
- So your maximum heart rate is 192bpm (beats per minute)

High intensity interval training or steady state cardio training

- For high intensity INTERVAL cardio training where you wish to burn fat and sustain lean muscle, note I said interval cardio, not steady state cardio where you move at a gradual and glacial pace consistently over a long period of time, then you should be aiming for 90% of your maximum heart rate for this to be most effective.
- If you are interested in low intensity steady state cardio just for fat loss purposes then aim for 60% as a beginner, 75% as an intermediate or anything above 75% for an advanced gym goer for this to be the most effective.

14 | MIND TO MUSCLE CONNECTION

This is one of the industry's biggest secrets.

How it's done: *Squeeze* for two to three seconds in order to achieve a peak contraction. That's it.

Sometimes we forget what we're actually doing at the gym because our mind wonders off about so many different things, and we move so fast through an exercise and the the entire workout, yet we continue to workout but we're not really working out, if you know what I mean. I refer to this as 'ghost training'. This behavior is counterproductive towards our goals. We need to be thinking about the muscle, essentially communicating with it. When performing an exercise you should be doing everything you can to *squeeze* the life out of that muscle group upon contraction, causing your mind to remember that sensation of that muscle being squeezed, which *then* causes you to squeeze that same muscle more frequently when you exercise, without really thinking about it.

Let me break this down a little bit more. Weight lifting tears your muscles fibers. That's how weight lifting stimulates muscle growth. It tears the muscle fibers deep within your muscles, and then your body repairs those muscle fibers while you sleep. That's why it's so important to get your full 7 to 8 hours of sleep a night after a workout. That's also why we wake up looking our best in the morning. Our muscles have regenerated and fibers have expanded during the night, making you look your best. This is where consistency in your routine comes in. Eat, sleep, train, and repeat. *Starting to make sense?*

A perfect example where mind to muscle connection is necessary is squat position. You don't squeeze your butt when you're lowering yourself to the ground with the weight on your shoulders because as you're lowering yourself you're not working anything just yet; you're only preparing the muscle for the work. Squeezing your butt muscles as you rise upwards in a squat position activates the different muscle groups in your butt (all three of them); this creates a mind to muscle memory. Your mind remembers to squeeze that muscle every time you're in the same position – strengthening that muscle. This is also how you switch muscles on or 'activate' them. It's also how you can make your pecs bounce or your butt cheeks bounce by learning to communicate with that muscle group. The harder the squeeze during your workouts, the more communication you have with that muscle, the more you're connecting with that muscle and the more you have control over it. If you don't feel anything when you're lifting then you are ghost training. Start squeezing those muscles and you will feel them tighten over time, realizing how much can control you actually have over them and their growth.

15 | TEMPO

Speed at which one repetition is performed is known as **tempo**.

The most beneficial tempo is denoted with 4 numbers i.e. 4-0-1-0.

Each of the 4 numbers is in seconds.

1. The first number represents the speed of the movement that follows one repetition
2. The second is the pause
3. The third is the action phase of the movement
4. The fourth is the pause

In the example of a bench press or a squat:

1. The first number denotes the speed at which the weight is lowered
2. The second is the pause at the bottom
3. The third is the speed at which he bar is pressed
4. And the fourth is the pause at the top

First off understand that the size of your muscles is dictated by the amount of tension you place on them. The more tension you place on your muscles, the more they'll grow. This is why it's so important to constantly increase the amount of weight and reps you do, because if you keep lifting the same amount of weight, it means you're constantly applying the same amount of tension on your muscles and thus they will remain the same size.

Put simply, a 4-0-1-0 tempo is:

- 1 second on the positive movement
- 4 seconds on the negative movement

With 0 second pauses at the top and bottom By going much slower on the negative movement, exploding on the positive, and not resting at the top or bottom, you're greatly increasing the amount of tension you place on your muscles.

16 | MY BUTT WORKOUT

This chapter includes explanations for beginners.

If you are an advanced or intermediate gym goer feel free to skip to the final chapter where you will find the workout without detail.

A notable mention:

- I have avoided using complex language i.e. gluteus medius, minimus and maximus, quadriceps and gastrocnemius, but instead butt, thighs and calves so it is easier for you to understand.

- Weight varies depending on your strength and capabilities. I recommend lifting what you can. I'm a firm believer in building up your strength over time. There's no rush. All you need to do is increase the weight after each set by at least 2.5-5kg for a beginner and anything greater than 10kg for an advanced weight lifter. You're not going to go home with any award or trophy for lifting 100kg on your first attempt. Sure, it's good for bragging points, but the purpose of this workout is to build your butt not hurt yourself so please be mindful of your weight choice!

Please also note:

- Locking your knees in any leg exercise can cause damage to your knees. Keep your knees 'soft'. Not wobbly in the slightest but 'soft' meaning when you reach the maximum range of a movement make sure your legs are not dead straight as this can damage the cartilage in your knees.
- With any butt workout, people tend to overarch their lower back. Keep a nice straight back and your pelvis tucked in when starting any movement on leg day. You can arch your back at another time in the mirror, but right now make sure your pelvis is sitting on a normal tilt and not poking out. There is no need to over-arch or hyper-extend your back when squatting. It's not the 'Anaconda' music video.

Definition of a 'superset':

- A superset is when you complete two exercises, intertwined together without stopping for a break. You only stop for a break after 1 set of each exercise is complete. So you do 1 for 1 then break, 2 for 2 then break, until all sets of each are complete. So you're basically doing 2 sets of 2 different movements back-to-back, breaking, then another 2. Make sure you are getting your rest between each superset otherwise you will fatigue quickly and burn out.

Let's begin!

1. Dynamic Stretching and Warm-Up

Start your butt workout with a few stretches. It doesn't matter what stretches you pick just get the blood flowing through your butt, hamstrings, calves, thighs, knees ankles and joints. Stretch for 3-4 minutes. Hold each stretch for 10 seconds. Dynamic stretches work effectively as a warm-up: high knees, side jumps, toe taps, etc.

2. Barbell Squats x Superset with Plated Squats

Equipment: Barbell squat rack

Muscle group: Butt, thighs, hamstrings

Sets: 4 sets, 45 seconds rest in between each

Repetitions: 12-15

Description: For this first exercise you will need a squat rack.

Load your squat rack with the lightest weight you can manage for your first set as for each set you will be increasing your weight based on your strength. Be aware that most barbells themselves weigh about 5-7kg alone. Perform 12 repetitions on the squat rack.

Superset: Step out of the squat rack, pick up a 5kg-10kg plate, step back and perform 10 plated squats. I use 20kg but that's because I've been doing this for a while. The plate should be held with both hands horizontally against your chest. Once the plated squats are complete, this is your first superset complete. So you've just done one set of barbell squats and one set of bodyweight squats back to back; otherwise known as a superset. Take a break for 45 seconds. Repeat 3 more times.

So in total you have 8 sets all together: 4 sets of barbell squats and 4 sets of singular plated squats. That's 8 sets in total with over 96 squats completed. That's a lot of squats for a beginner. You don't need to complete them all; you can reduce your sets down to 3 barbell squats and 3 sets of singular plated squats so 6 sets in total. Take your time and don't feel pressured. Ease your way into it.

If you still feel like 6 sets is a lot, you can break it down even more to 3 sets of singular plated squats alone without the 3 sets of barbell squats. That's absolutely fine. That's just 3 sets, which is a standard number for a beginner. You should be getting a feel and understanding of what your body can do and manage. After all, you have another 9-10 exercises to go, so you don't want to fatigue your body just squatting. But this is the workout that I've done for the past few years by building my strength. It just takes time and practice

3. Dumbbell Deadlift x Superset with Walking Dumbbell Lunges

Equipment: Dumbbells

Muscle group: Hamstrings

Sets: 3 sets, 45 seconds rest in between each

Repetitions: 12-14

Description: Position two 20kg plates on the ground side by side. Step your toes on to each one of them separating your feet so they are shoulder width apart – the plates being large in size should give you enough room when you step your toes on to the edges, creating space between your legs. Your toes should be aligned with your shoulders. Pick up two dumbbells and hold them with your backhand facing frontwards where your toes are pointing. The dumbbells should be positioned horizontal now against your thighs. Slowly push your butt outwards (without arching) and bend down at your hips bringing the dumbbells down along your legs. The pushing out of the butt and the descent with the barbells down to your toes along your legs should happen simultaneously. So as soon as you push out, you should have already started travelling the dumbbells down your legs. Your dumbbell should be an inch or two away from your legs so they don't move forwards. Go as low as you can go towards your toes, hold for two seconds and come back up.

Superset: After 1 set of your deadlifts are done, use the same dumbbells and stand back aside and perform 12 walking body lunges on each leg. That's 1 superset complete. Break. Then complete 2 more sets.

Sets: 3

Repetitions: 12

4. Lying Hamstring Curls

Equipment: Lying leg curl machine

Muscle group: Hamstrings

Sets: 3 sets, 30 seconds rest in between each

Repetitions: 15-20

Description: Lie down on your stomach on an angled leg curl machine, keeping your chest flat against the padding and tucking your legs under the cylinder padding. Grip your hands on the handles below the machine, if there is no handles grip the side of the padding where your head hangs over. Squeezing your butt cheeks together and your hamstrings, lift your legs up all the way with your toes pointing out. Don't squeeze through your toes as that puts pressure on your ankles. Focus on squeezing your hamstrings and your butt. You will feel a pinch behind your knees as well. This is OK and works in conjunction with your hamstrings. The key here is not to arch your back and not to squeeze your actual feet but your entire leg, as well as butt.

5. Leg Press x Superset with Hack Squat

Equipment: Leg press machine

Muscle group: Butt, thighs, hamstrings

Sets: 3 sets, 45 seconds rest in between each

Repetitions: 12-15

Description: This is fantastic for growing your butt as it takes the stress off the back unlike most leg exercises and redirects it to the hamstrings, thighs, and most importantly, your butt! You want to adjust the seat as close as possible horizontally to the platform where the feet are placed. This will allow the movement to be as deep as possible. The deeper the movement, the more it will target the glutes. Make sure you place your feet as high as possible vertically on the platform. The higher your feet, the more your body will rely on your butt to do the work. The lower your feet, the more your thighs will feel the movement. When you undo the lever, grip the side of your seat and lower your legs as close as possible to your chest. When pushing upwards to starting position squeeze your glutes as hard as possible. As you're lifting the weight, press your knees together as you do each repetition. This will cause your butt to squeeze together making them firmer and tighter, as well as working the muscles of the inner thigh.

Superset: After 1 set of your leg press is complete; move over to the hack squat to perform 10-12 hack squats at a substantially lightweight. The weight doesn't have to be heavy as this is pretty much a leg press only standing; you're just changing the circulation of blood flow and the direction in which your muscles are pushing towards. The leg press, you're pushing upwards, and hack squat you're pushing downwards – which I find extremely helpful with building a bigger butt as you're getting a wholesome workout that activates all your glute muscles at different angles and positions. After your hack squats are complete, that's 1 superset complete. Have a 45 second rest. Then complete 2 more sets.

Sets: 3

Repetitions: 10-12

6. Leg Extensions x Superset with Jump Squats

Equipment: Seated leg extension machine

Muscle group: Thighs

Sets: 3 sets, 45 seconds rest in between each

Repetitions: 12-15

Description: Make yourself comfortable on the seat and ensure that your body is positioned at a 90-degree angle. When extending your legs, ensure that the rest of your body remains still on the seat so avoid using your whole body to force your legs upwards. The point is to use your legs. Some people squeeze so hard on the grip of their chair or bend forward in the seat to be able to lift their legs up, which puts strain on your back. Do not lock your knees at the top, meaning keep them slightly bent when you reach the highest positioning you can.

Superset: After 1 set of your seated leg extensions are complete; step aside and perform 12-15 body weight jump squats with your hands softly behind your ears/head – similar the same position where they would be when you're doing crunches or sit ups on the ground. It will be tricky to balance if you have never done this before because you're hands aren't balancing you, they're behind your ears, but try a few attempts without the jump to and then incorporate the jump once you've got the balance. Soft jump, nothing high and major, just enough to lift off the ground. After your jump squats are complete, that's 1 superset complete. Have a 45 second rest. Then complete 2 more sets.

Sets: 3

Repetitions: 12-15

7. Standing Calf Raises

Equipment: Standing calf raise machine or on a smith machine

Muscle group: Calves

Sets: 4 sets, 30 seconds rest in between each

Repetitions: 15-20

Description: Step onto the platform, gripping your hands on to the handlebars, head between the padding and resting on your shoulders. Make sure you to keep your back straight with a slight bend at the knees. If your gym doesn't have a standing calf raise machine, you can use the smith machine and place a step up (every gym should have these) on the ground and step your toes on to the edge. Lift up from your toes feeling the pinch in your calves and return slowly, without letting the weight hit the weight stack. As it's only a toe raise, if done quickly and without a proper tempo, you will feel nothing. The key is to squeeze when your toes have lifted the weight and your calves are contracting. Hold for 3-4 seconds. Make sure you are getting a full range of motion when you rise from your toes then return to your starting height.

8. Kettlebell Hip Thrusts

Equipment: Kettlebell and flat bench

Muscle group: Butt

Sets: 3 sets, 30 seconds rest in between each

Repetitions: 15-20

Description: Positioning yourself correctly here will be a bit tricky for a beginner. The position of your upper to mid back should be on the edge of a flat bench with both feet firmly on the ground. Your whole back should not be resting on the bench; you should just be leaning off the bench using your upper to mid back only. Your body should be at a 90-degree angle if we are looking at the angle from your legs to the ground. Feet should be firmly on the ground with a bit of distance between them. Now bring the kettlebell off the floor and gently place it on your lower pelvis with the handle facing your body and the round part facing your lower body. Hold the kettlebell carefully, and thrust upwards bringing your hips as high as possible. Hold the position, and squeeze all your butt muscles for 3-4 seconds. Slowly lower your hips back down without touching the ground, just relaxing your hips, and rest for a second, and then repeat the exercise. The hip thrust is very stable and simple to perform. I know this movement is popular with a barbell across your lap or a dumbbell, but I feel this is can get a bit tricky and tends to be difficult to put on top of yourself. Hip thrusts maximize tension on the glutes and do a better job of hitting the upper fibers, giving you that shelf-like booty.

9. One-Legged Cable Kick Backs

Equipment: Cable machine

Muscle group: Butt

Sets: 3

Repetitions: 15-20

Description: Hook an ankle cuff to a low cable pulley and then attach the cuff to your ankle. Face the weight stack from a distance of about two feet (half a meter), grasping the steel frame for support. Your whole body should be aligned with the weight stack and your other leg that is not strapped to a cuff should be positioned firmly on the ground. Now what you do is tilt at the pelvis slightly while both hands are gripping either on to the metal pole of the cable machine (be careful not to get your fingers caught in the cable – some machines have handle bars for these movements, but older machines do not so you need to carefully decide where to place your hands). Your tilt should be about 45 degrees, definitely not 90 as this is not helpful. Once you're tilted forward, kick your leg that is strapped as high as in can go in a backwards kicking motion. If you've never done this it might take a bit to get used to. The key is to hold and squeeze when your leg is high in the air. If you just kick your leg forwards and backwards you wont feel a thing. Kick, hold, squeeze and return. Pause. And repeat. While keeping your knees and hips bent slightly and your abs tight, contract your glutes to slowly kick the working leg back as high as it will comfortably go as you breathe out. Now slowly bring your working leg forward, relaxing the cable until you reach the starting position.

10. Cable Pull Through

Equipment: Cable machine

Muscle group: Butt

Sets: 3

Repetitions: 15-20

Description: Using the rope handle of the cable machine, which is very easy, to spot it's usually a thick rope-like looking device, you want to face away from the machine with the rope on the bottom level of the cable machine. Now make a small distance with your legs almost shoulder width apart. Bend down and grab the handles of the rope with both hands so each hand should be holding a piece of the rope. Start at a position here you are bent downwards, causing the rope and cable to retract into the machine. Now rise upwards from the hips thrusting forward while squeezing your butt! This might look a bit funny to others but you will be laughing at the haters when your butt is plumper after this workout and who cares what they think! Repeat the movement. Bend, and thrust. Bend and snap!

11. Cool down: Stairmaster

I conclude my butt workout sessions with 15 minutes on the Stairmaster as detailed in chapter 13: *The Truth Behind Cardio.*

17 | MY BUTT WORKOUT

The Formula for a bigger, rounder, perkier and more defined butt:

Warm-up: Dynamic stretching

1. Barbell Squats x Superset with Plated Squats
2. Dumbbell Deadlift x Superset with Walking Dumbbell Lunges
3. Lying Hamstring Curls
4. Leg Press x Superset with Hack Squat
5. Leg Extensions x Superset with Jump Squats
6. Standing Calf Raises
7. Kettlebell Hip Thrusts
8. One-Legged Cable Kick Backs
9. Cable Pull Through
10. Cool down: Stairmaster

Congratulations!

You have now reached the end of *The Formula.*

I most excited to see your goals come to life. A photo can last a lifetime; therefore I encourage all my readers to send me any before and after pictures of their choosing displaying their hard work to document their journey and goals achieved with the help of *The Formula.* You will also be featured on my Instagram and website.

Don't ever feel ashamed to share your achievements with the world.

For any other enquiries: contact@eliasnohraofficial.com
or feel free to leave a message on Instagram.

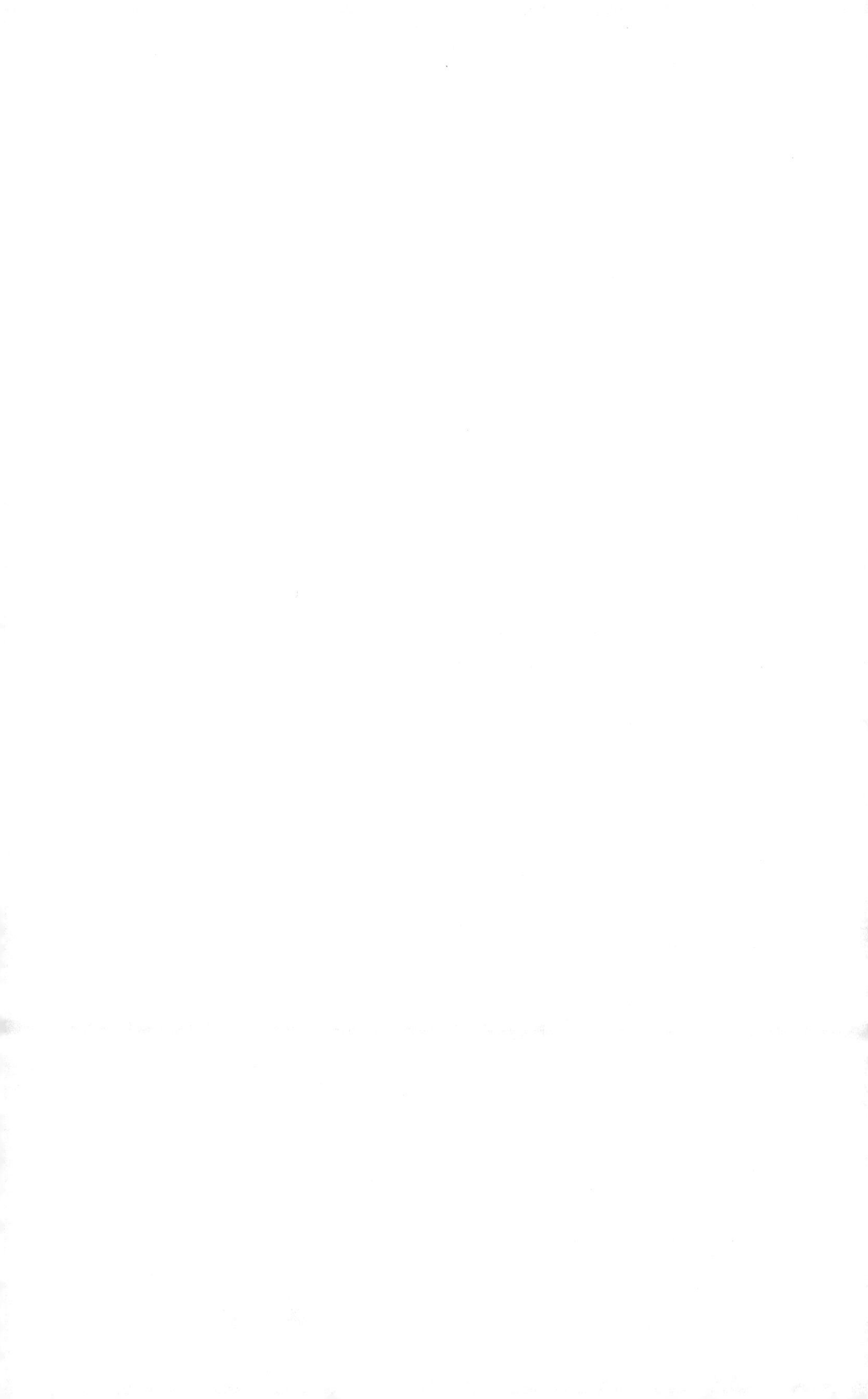

Made in the USA
Middletown, DE
28 June 2018